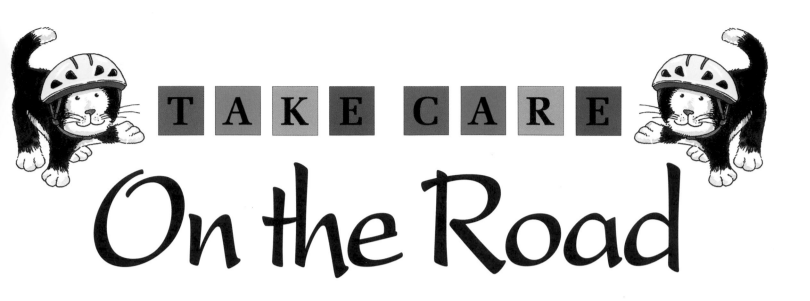

TAKE CARE
On the Road

Carole Wale

RoSPA

Photographer: Angus Blackburn

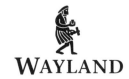

WAYLAND

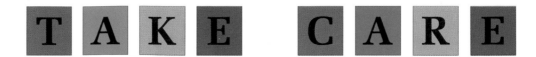

At Home   On Your Own
Near Water   On the Road

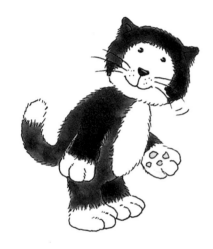

Editor: Katie Orchard
Designer: Jean Wheeler
Artist: Lynne Farmer
Production controller: Carol Titchener

First published in 1996 by Wayland Publishers Ltd
61 Western Road, Hove,
East Sussex BN3 1JD
England

British Library Cataloguing in Publication Data
Wale, Carole
Take Care On the Road. – (Take Care series)
I. Title II. Series
363.125

ISBN 0 7502 1785 5

Typeset by Jean Wheeler, in England
Printed and bound in England by B.P.C Paulton Books

Contents

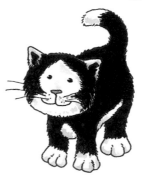

The words that appear in **bold** are explained in the picture glossary on page 30.

Holding Hands

Take care when you are out and about. Always take an adult with you.

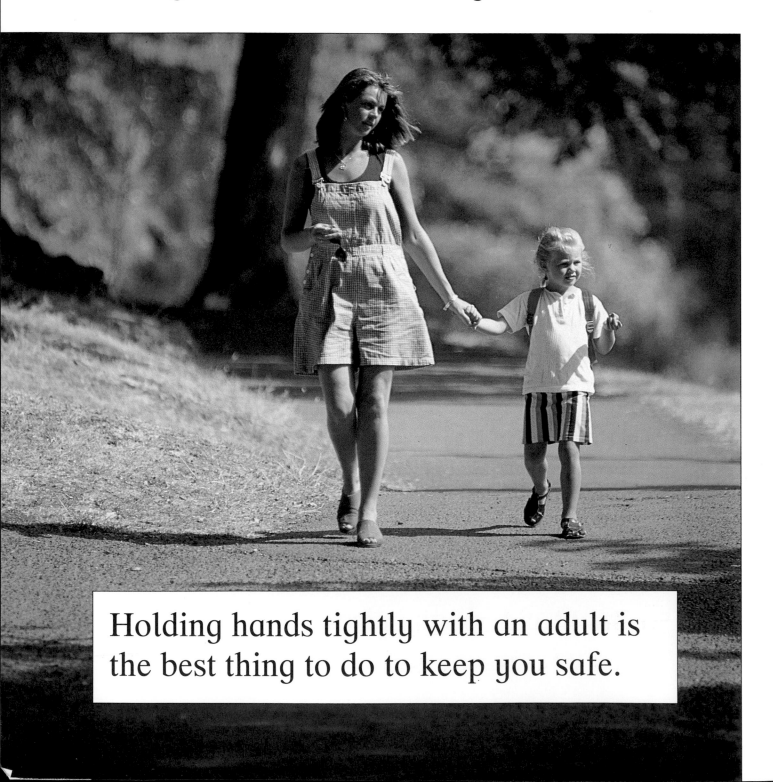

Holding hands tightly with an adult is the best thing to do to keep you safe.

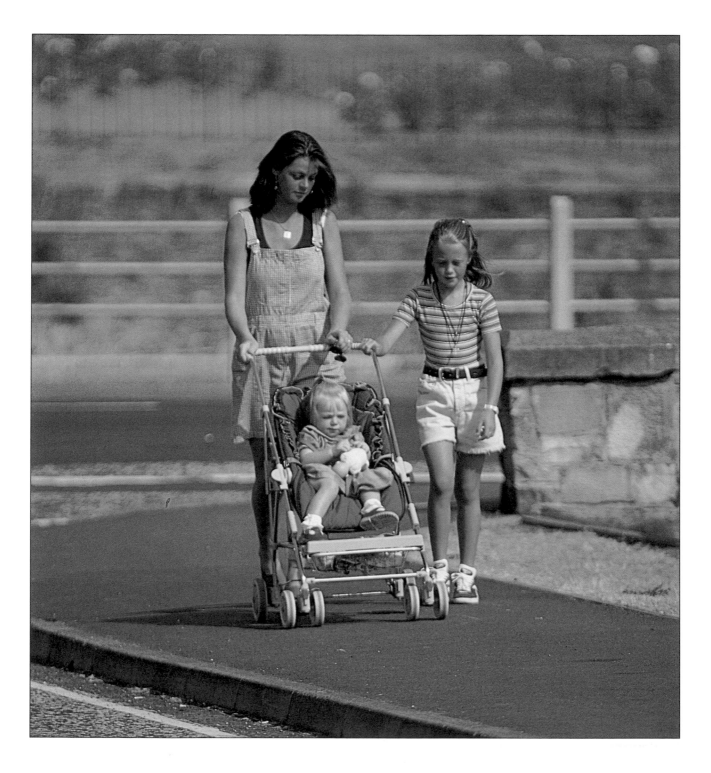

If you can't hold someone's hand, hold on to the handle of a shopping bag or the handlebars of a pushchair.

Pavements are for People

Pavements are special places where it is safe for people to walk. People who walk on pavements are called pedestrians.

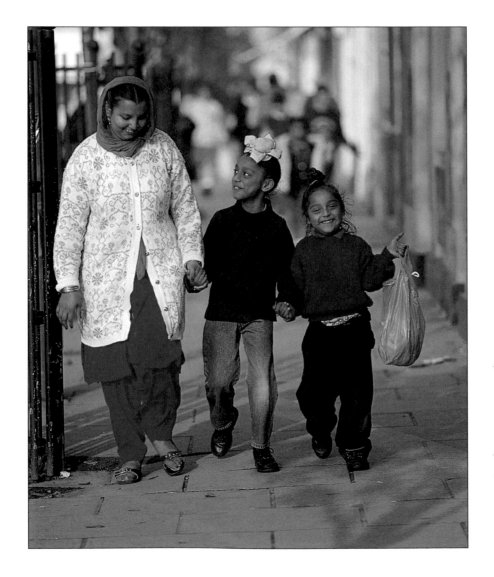

Walk on the inside of the pavement, away from the kerb.

Sometimes, vehicles have to cross the pavement to get in or out of **driveways**.

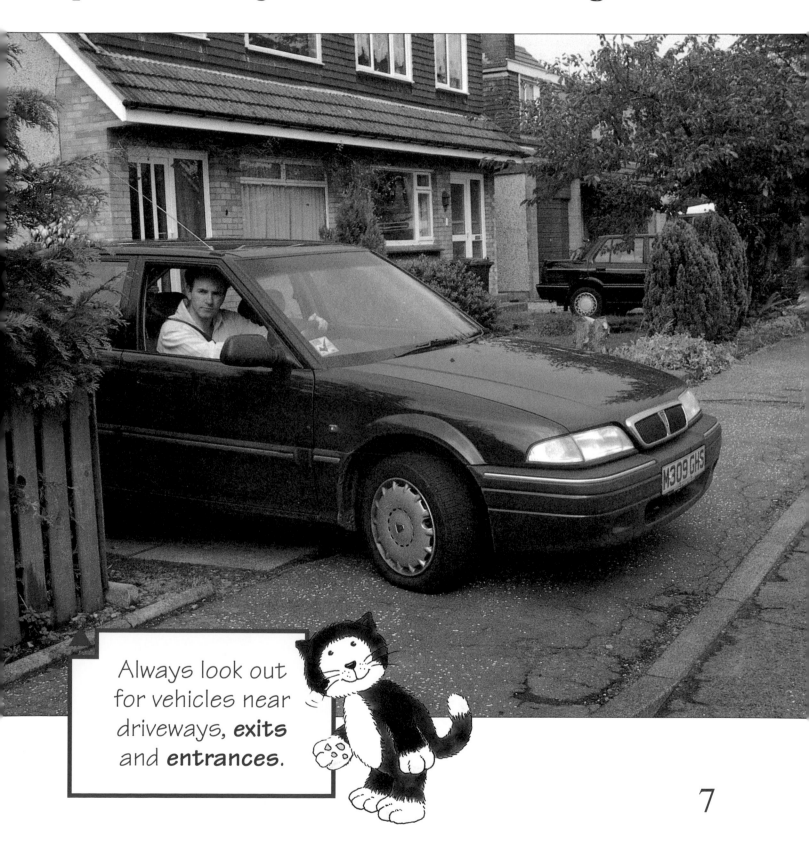

Always look out for vehicles near driveways, **exits** and **entrances**.

7

Roads are for Vehicles

Roads are special places for vehicles. Vehicles have wheels and are big, heavy and fast. They travel much faster than people.

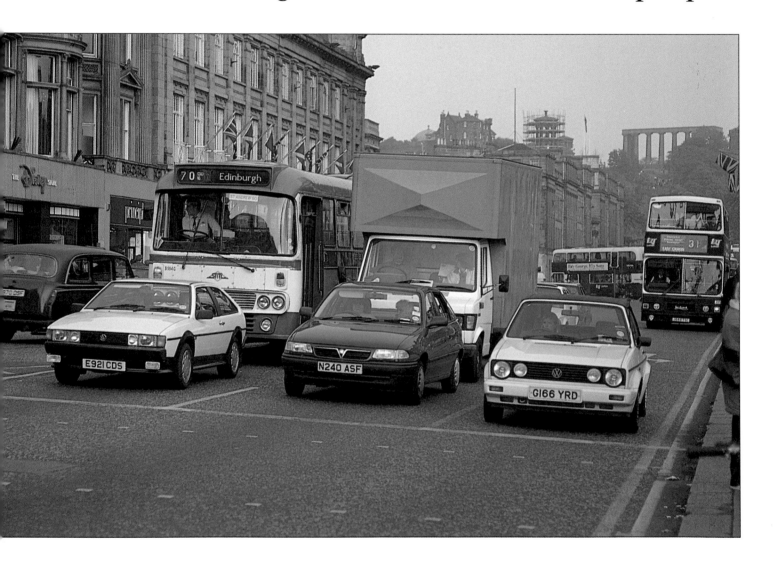

The cars, truck, buses and taxi in this picture are all vehicles.

Motorbikes are vehicles too.
Vehicles move together along roads. This
is called traffic.

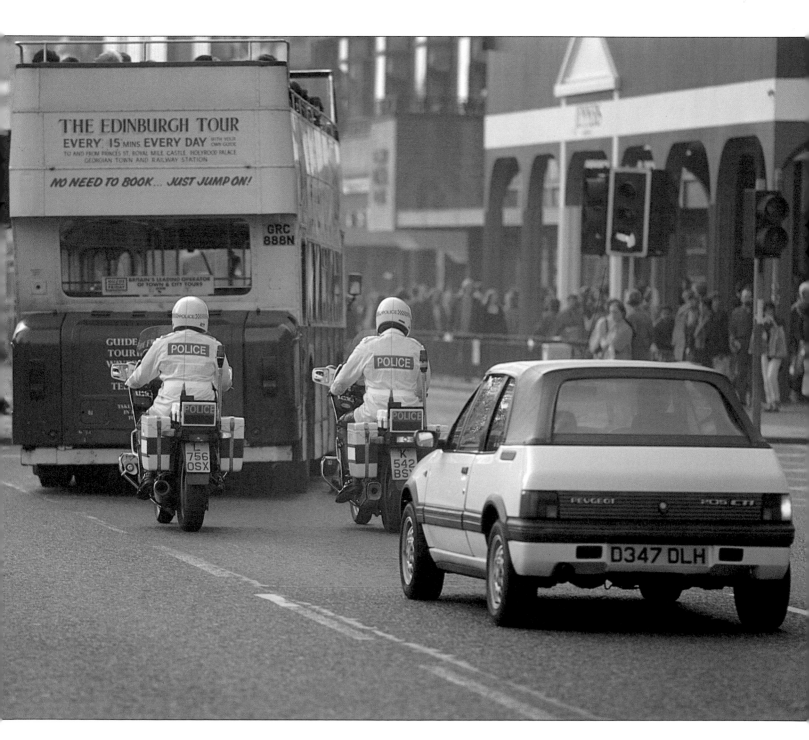

In the Street

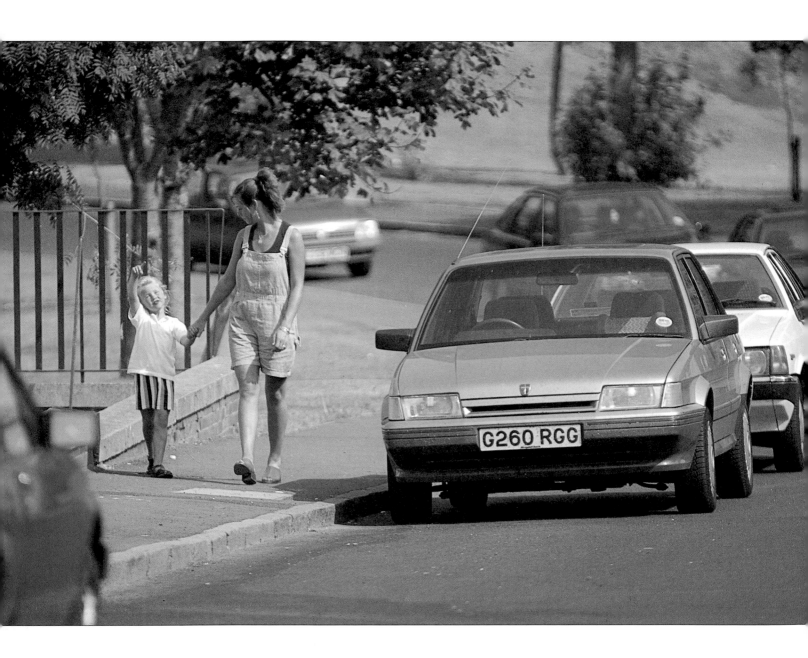

A street is the name for a road in a town. When you are in a street you must walk along the pavement and hold hands with an adult.

Look at this busy street with its shops, road signs and **pelican crossing**.

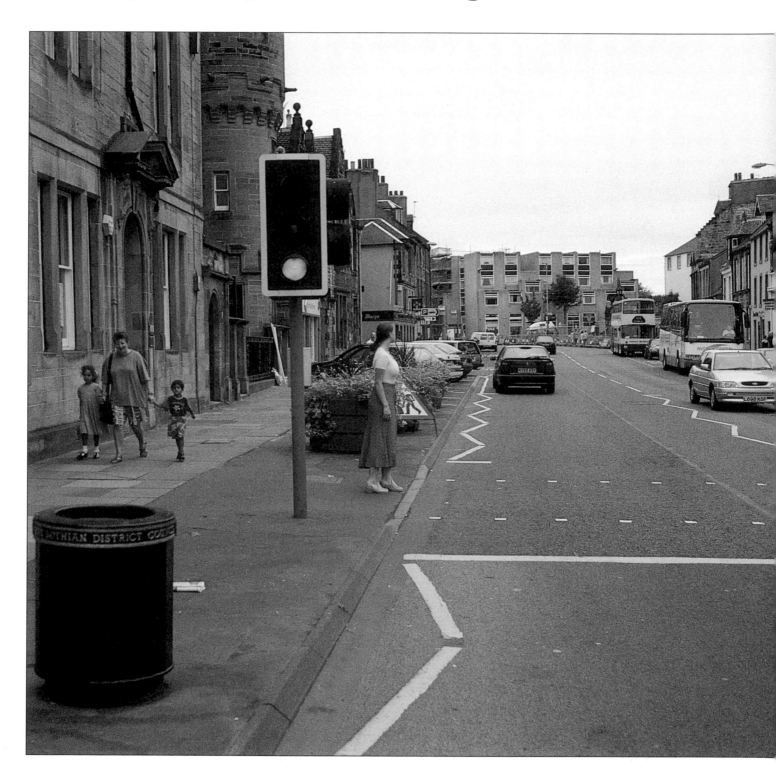

Stop!

Stop at the kerb when you want to cross the road. Keep your feet together while you look and listen for traffic.

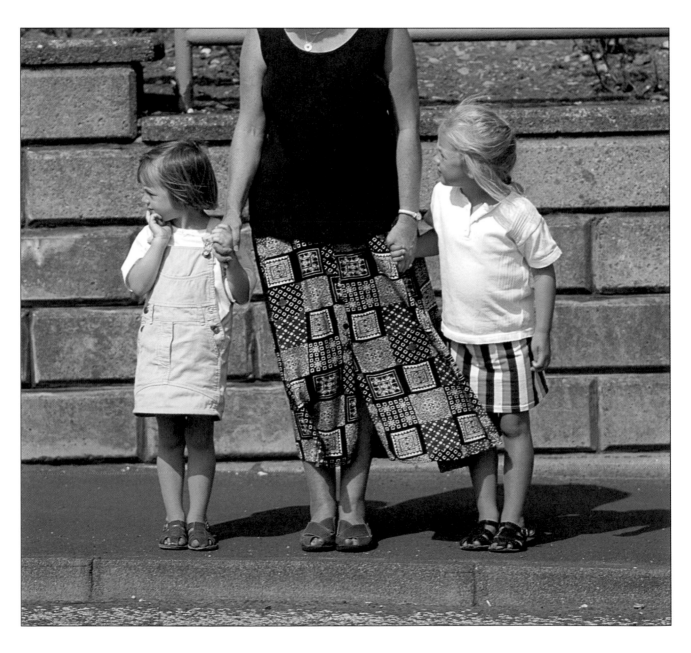

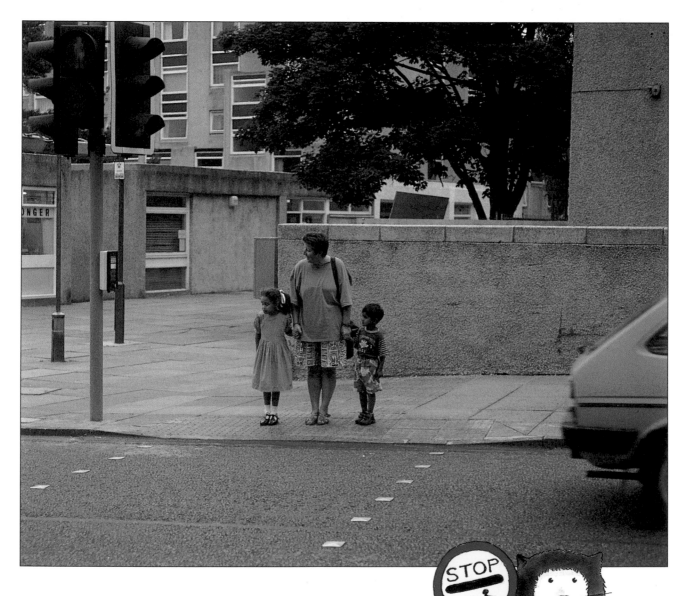

At the pelican crossing, stop and wait when the red person is showing. Cross only when the steady green person is showing; do not start to cross if it is flashing.

When there is no crossing, stop and wait at the kerb with an adult until it is safe to cross.

Look!

Look all around for traffic. Keep looking
as you cross the road.

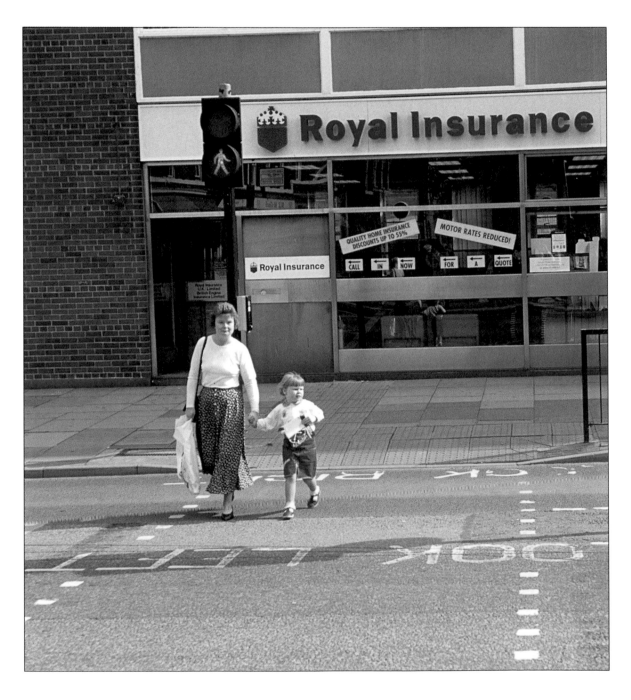

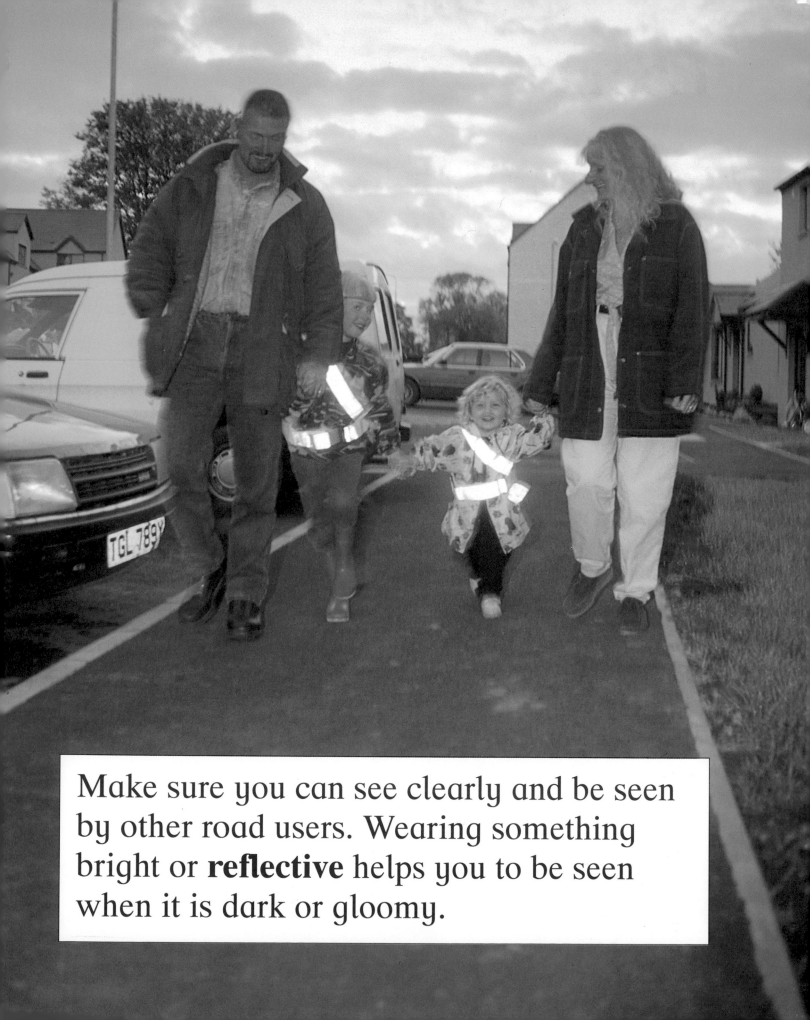

Make sure you can see clearly and be seen by other road users. Wearing something bright or **reflective** helps you to be seen when it is dark or gloomy.

Listen!

Listen carefully for traffic sounds when you cross the road. Keep listening as you cross.

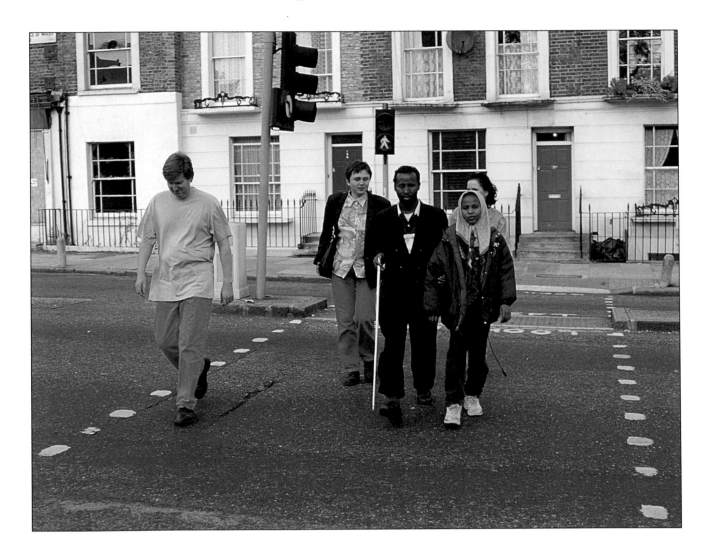

The pelican crossing makes a bleeping sound when it is safe to cross. This helps blind people cross the road.

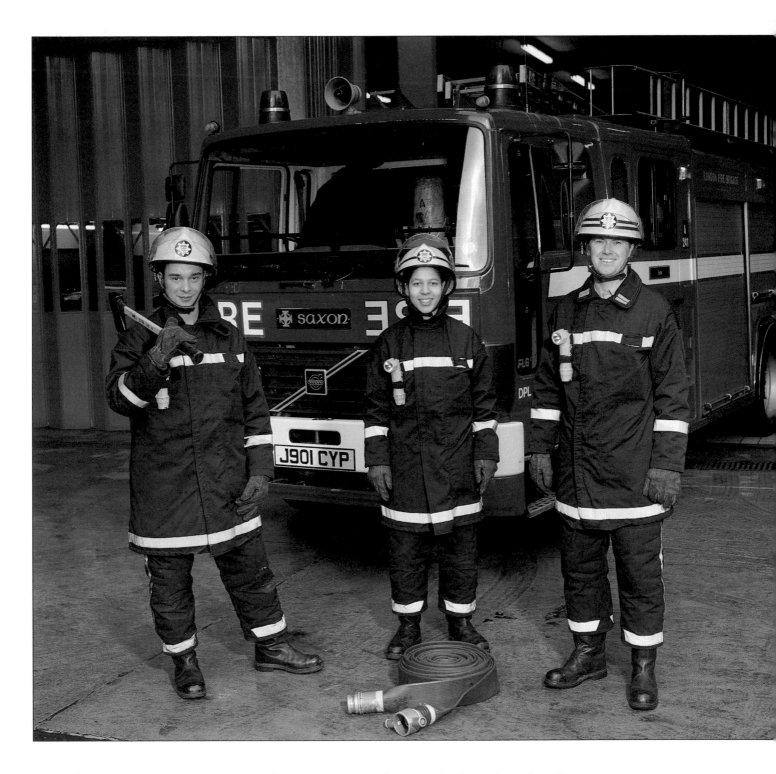

Vehicles can make sounds with their horns
to warn us that they are there. **Emergency
vehicles** like this fire engine have loud sirens.

Helping Us Cross the Road

The **school crossing patrol** has a sign that tells drivers to stop so you can cross the road safely.

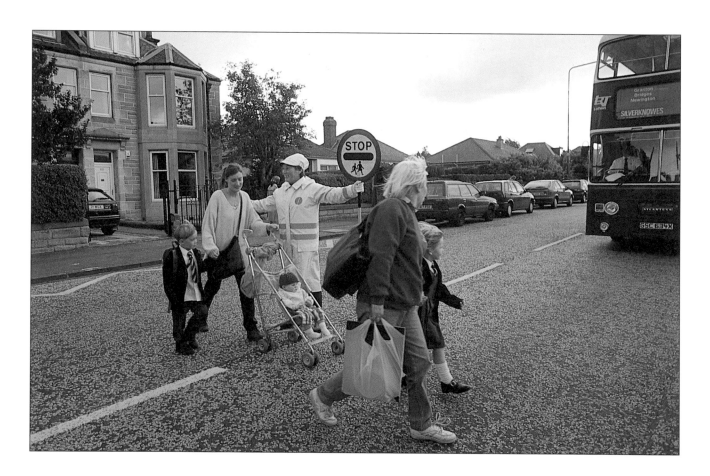

Other people who can help you cross the road are your parents, teachers, police and **traffic wardens**.

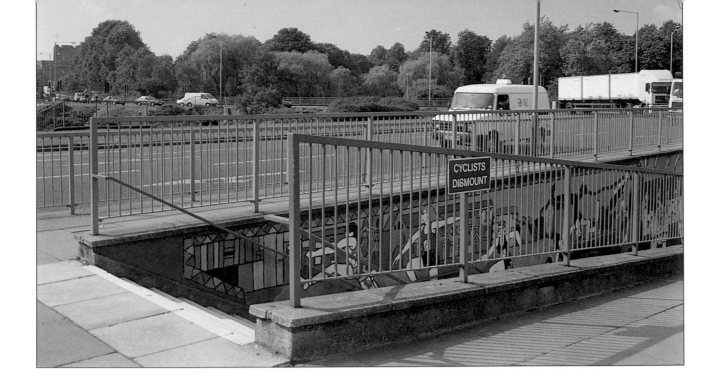

Good places to cross are at **subways** ▲, **zebra crossings** ▼, pelican crossings and **foot-bridges**.

Always find a good place to cross the road away from parked cars, bends, corners and hills. ▲

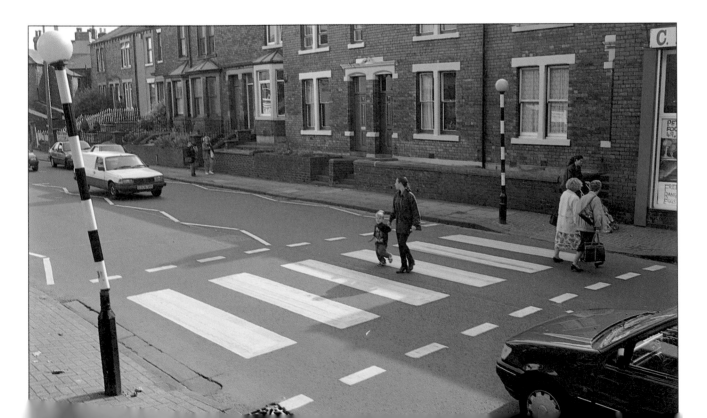

Quiet Roads and Busy Roads

There are many different types of roads.
Some roads are busy, like high streets.
Watch out for fast-moving traffic
on city roads.

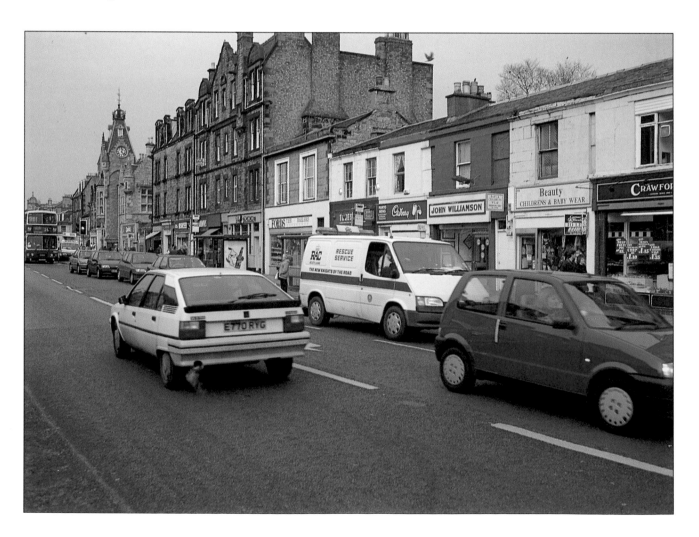

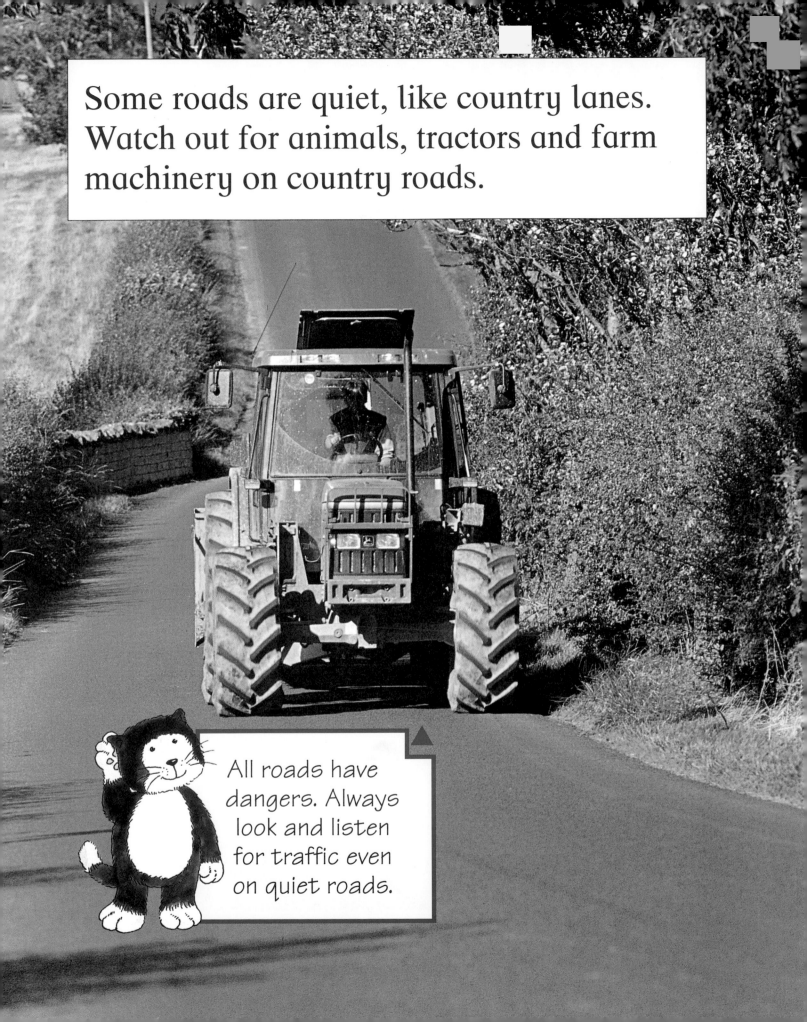

Some roads are quiet, like country lanes. Watch out for animals, tractors and farm machinery on country roads.

All roads have dangers. Always look and listen for traffic even on quiet roads.

Travelling by Car

Be a safe passenger. Get in and out of the car on the side nearest to the pavement.

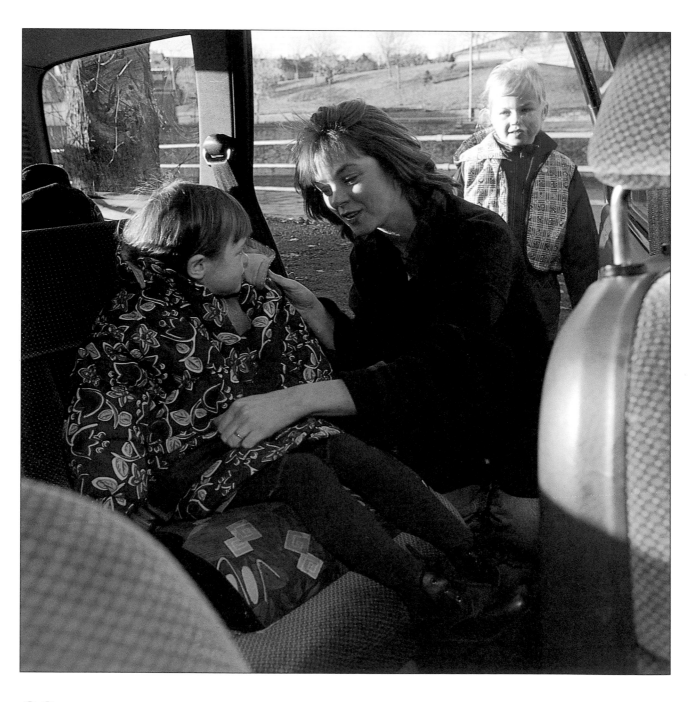

Sit in the back seat of the car and wear a seat belt. Younger children need a **booster seat** to keep them safe.

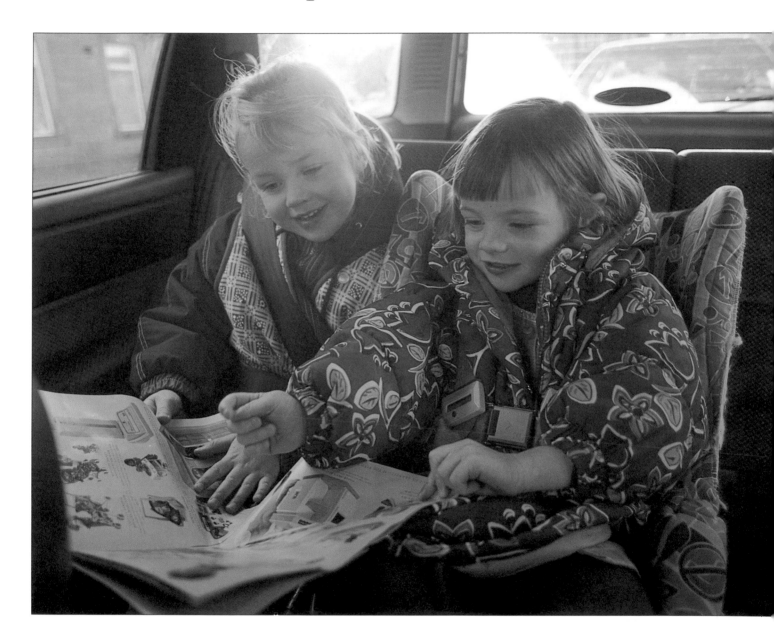

Find something quiet to do during the journey so that you don't disturb the driver.

Travelling by Bus

Take care at the bus stop. Stand well back while you wait for the bus. Let people get off the bus before you try to get on.

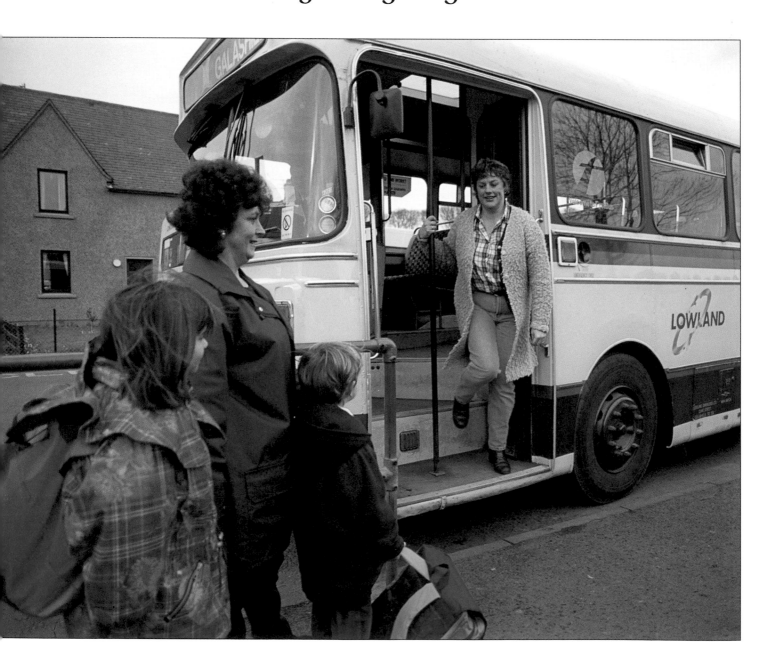

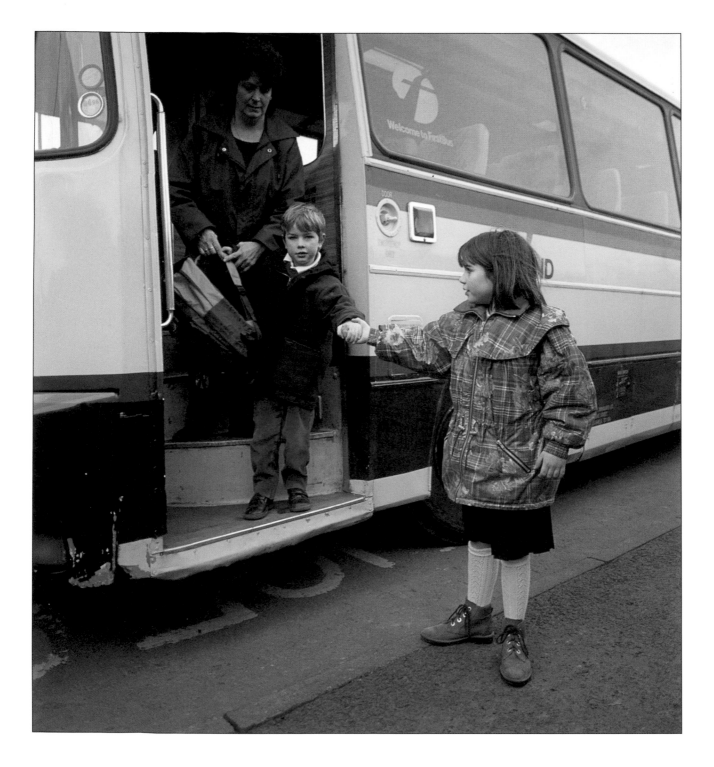

Wait for the bus to stop before you try to get off. Let the bus move away before you try to cross the road with an adult.

Learning to Cycle

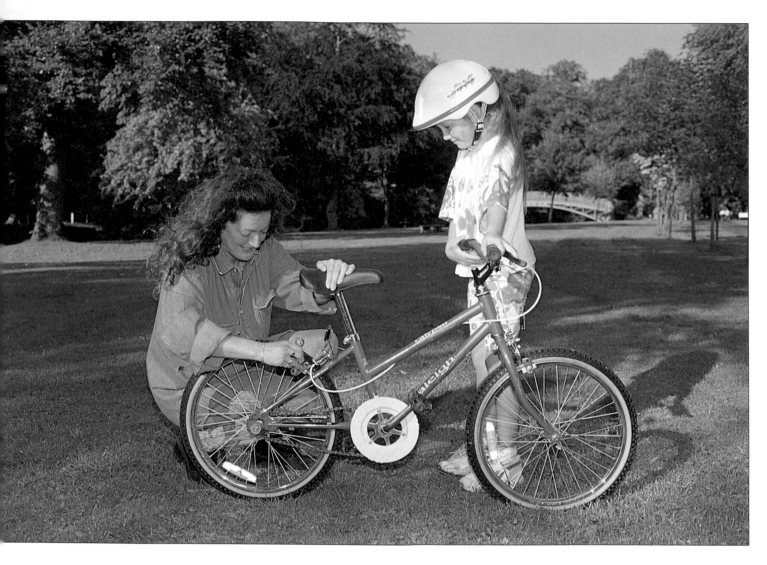

Ask an adult to make sure that your saddle is at the right height for you.

Always wear a **safety helmet** when you cycle. Sit properly in the saddle and pedal with the **balls of your feet**.

Practise riding your bike in a safe place like a park or a playground. Make sure you have an adult to watch you.

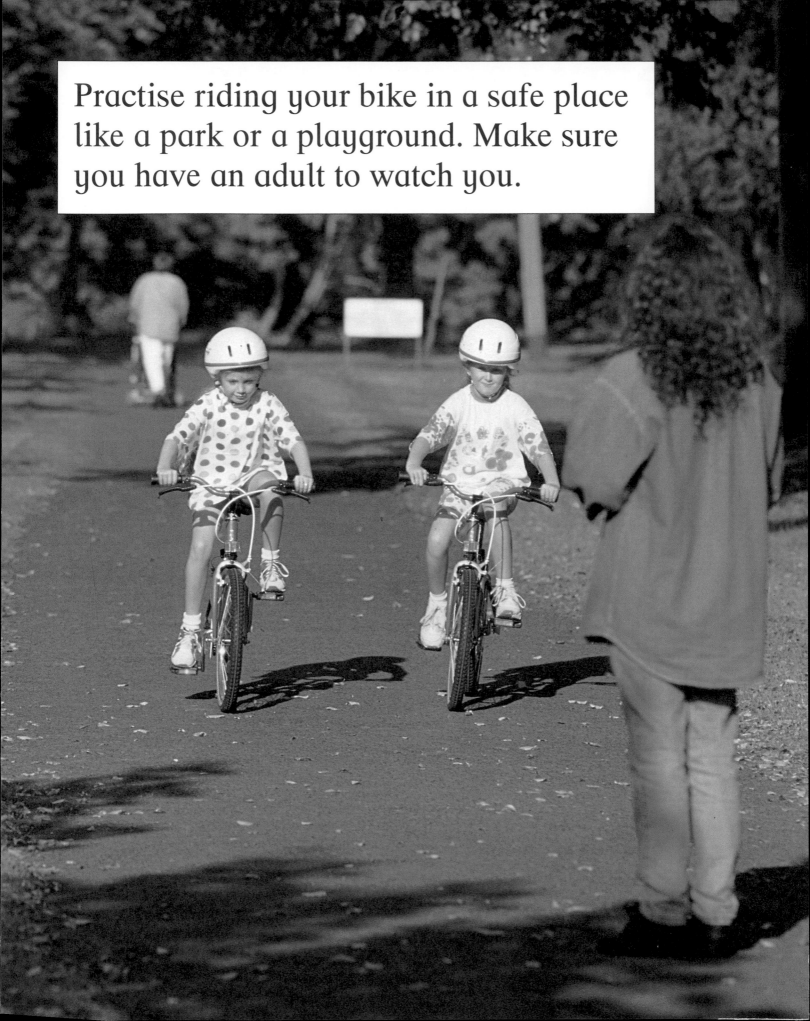

Safe Places to Play

Play in a safe place like the garden, park or playground. Make sure that you have an adult to watch over you.

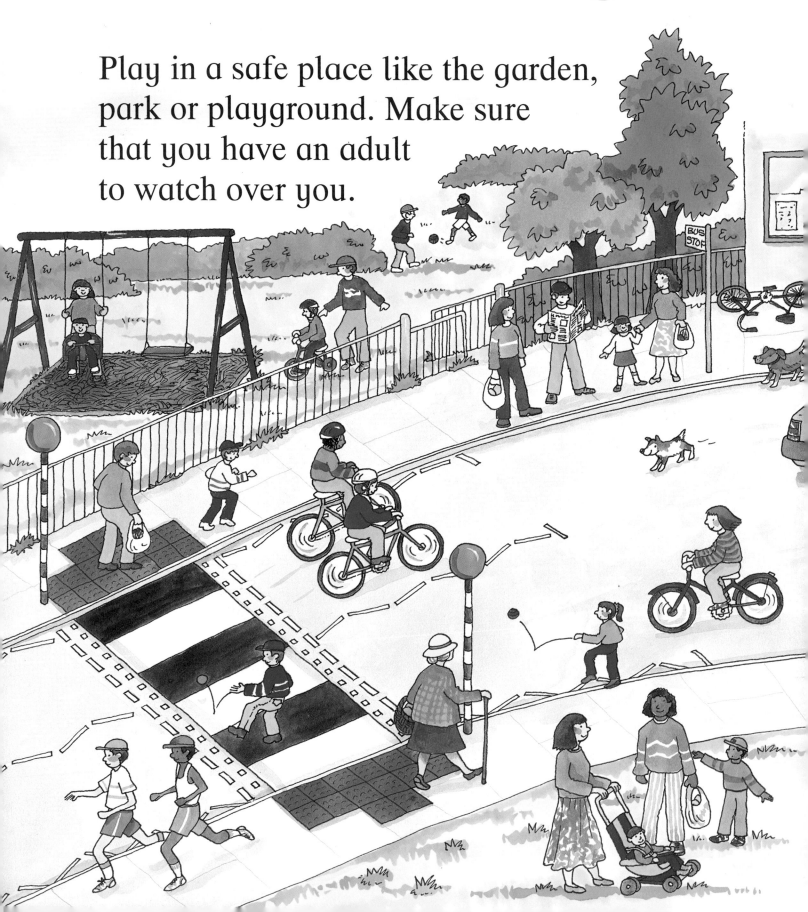

Roads and pavements are not safe places to play. Always take care when you are playing outside.

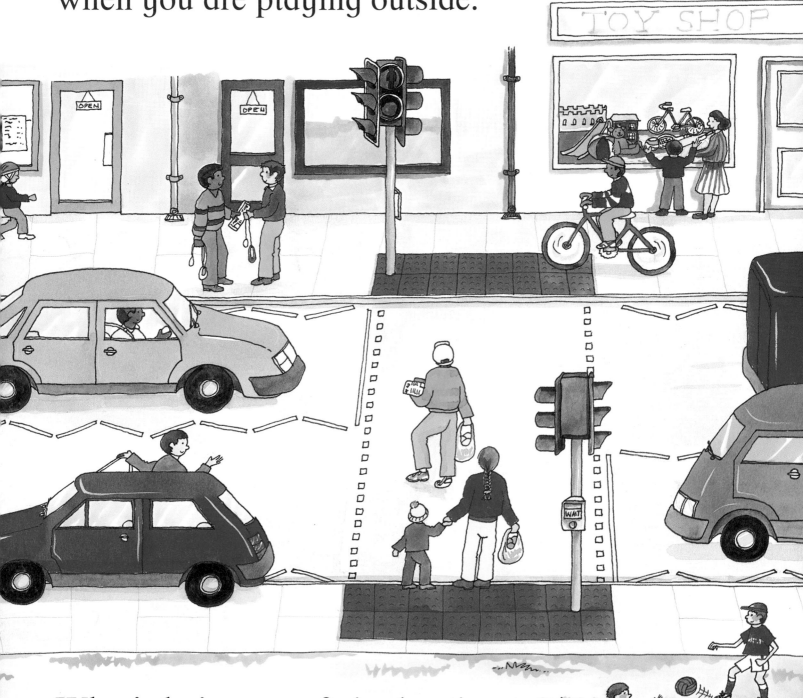

Who is being unsafe in the picture?
Who is being safe?
(Answers on page 30.)

Picture Glossary

 balls of your feet The bottoms of your feet, just behind your toes.

 booster seat A raised safety seat for a small child.

 driveways Private paths or small roads leading to houses or other buildings.

 emergency vehicles Vehicles such as ambulances, police cars and fire engines.

 entrance An opening off a road leading into a place or building.

 exit An opening leading from a place or building on to the road.

 foot-bridges Special bridges that pedestrians use to walk safely over busy roads.

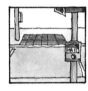 **pelican crossing** Where you press a button to work a signal which tells the traffic to stop.

 reflective Something that shines brightly in headlights or street lights when it is dark.

 safety helmet A special hard hat that protects your head if you fall off your bicycle.

 school crossing patrol He or she carries a large, round sign that tells the traffic to stop.

 subways Special tunnels under busy roads for people to walk through safely.

 traffic wardens People whose job it is to watch out for cars that are not parked safely.

 zebra crossings Crossings with black and white stripes painted on the road.

Answers to pages 28–9: Unsafe people include: the children playing with balls near a road, the car driver parking his car on the pavement and getting out on the road side, the cyclists without safety helmets, the man crossing the road without waiting for the green-lit man, and the dog-owners letting their dogs off the lead on a busy street. Safe people include: the children with adults in the park, people on bicycles wearing safety helmets, the child and mother holding hands and waiting at the pelican crossing, and the child and mother holding hands at the bus stop.

Books to Read

Be Safe On the Road by Pete Sanders (Franklin Watts, 1989)

Crossing Roads by Althea (Dinosaur Publications, 1988)

Look Out On the Road by Helena Ramsay (Red Rainbows, Evans Brothers Ltd, 1994)

Roads by Kate Petty and Terry Cash (A&C Black, 1990)

Stay Safe! by Anne Qualter and John Quinn (Wayland, 1993)

Watch Out! On the Road by Elizabeth Clark (Wayland, 1991)

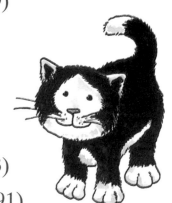

Notes for Parents and Teachers

Parents and teachers have a crucial role to play in helping children develop safety skills and good road safety habits. Children like to imitate adult behaviour, so set a good example.

Young children should not attempt to cross roads by themselves. Their small stature and lack of experience make them easy targets for road accidents.

Always hold the child's hand firmly when going out into the road, or let the child hold on to a bag or the handlebars of a pushchair.

Emphasize the importance of 'Stop, Look and Listen' and practise it frequently. Children can begin to learn the Green Cross Code in the context of real road situations.

Make sure your child has something light and bright to wear at night and in bad weather. Have something reflective for night and fluorescent for daytime.

Only use safe places to cross the road such as pedestrian crossings, subways and foot-bridges. Involve the child by talking through each situation.

Parked cars can be a problem. Avoid crossing between parked cars with young children. Where there is no choice, treat the edge of the cars as a kerb. Help children recognize when a car is about to move off.

Help children become safe passengers. Give them something to do on journeys and explain why drivers need to concentrate on the road. In cars, the safest place for any child is in the back seat wearing a properly designed restraint such as a special car seat or booster cushion and seat belt. Children should sit with you on buses. Always wait until a bus has moved away from the bus stop before crossing the road with a child.

Make sure your child's bicycle is a suitable size for their age and build. Make regular checks of the tyres, brakes and steering. Children under nine should practise riding in safe places like parks or playgrounds. At around nine, children can take the cyclist training. Only buy a cycle helmet that meets a recognized safety standard. Once a helmet has been damaged, make sure that it is replaced.

Encourage children to think about the safety needs of others such as the deaf and blind.

For more information about road safety education, write to: The Safety Education Department, RoSPA, Edgbaston Park, 353 Bristol Road, Birmingham, B5 7ST. Alternatively, contact your local road safety officer who can help you with all aspects of road safety.

Index

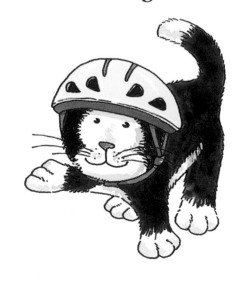